THE TLC DIET COOKBOOK

FOR

NEWBIES AND BEGINNERS

BY

Dr. Christen Zimmermann

Table of Contents

INTRODUCTION

The Therapeutic Lifestyle Changes diet, or TLC diet, was created by the National Institutes of Health. It's designed for people who want to make heart-healthy diet and exercise choices. With millions of people at risk of cardiovascular disease, the TLC diet emphasizes the use of nutrition and exercise as a first-line approach to disease prevention.

For more than a decade, health experts have regarded the TLC diet as one of the healthiest methods to reduce cholesterol levels and improve heart health. The diet seeks to eradicate unhealthy habits, such as poor dietary choices and a sedentary lifestyle. Followers of the TLC diet aim for specific calorie and macronutrient intakes depending on their sex and health goals. Though the premise of the program is centered on improving heart health, some people also follow it to lose weight.

WHAT YOU NEED TO KNOW

The TLC diet is divided into three components: diet, physical activity, and weight management. The program recommends 30 minutes of moderate-intensity exercise to promote weight management. Followers should aim to exercise most days of the week, if not every day. Both diet and physical activity contribute to healthy weight management. According to medical experts, being overweight or obese increases the risk of high cholesterol, high blood pressure, diabetes, heart disease, and more.3 The TLC diet encourages people to make an effort to reach a healthy weight to further decrease the risk of serious health problems.

The TLC diet also emphasizes eating behaviors more so than the time of day meals are consumed. For example, the program advises against eating dinner or snacking while watching TV, as this can lead to overeating. You can also practice slowing down your eating to give your brain more time to register fullness.

Pros

Encourages Healthy Lifestyle Habits

The TLC diet isn't a quick fix or fad diet. It's a combination of healthy lifestyle changes that can be sustained long-term to improve overall health.

While the focus is primarily on heart-healthy food, the TLC diet also makes an effort to encourage followers to exercise regularly. Other healthy lifestyle habits promoted on the TLC diet include drinking enough water, eating slower, and reading nutrition facts labels.

Incorporates Nutrient-Dense Whole Foods

In order to lose weight, you must consume fewer calories than you're burning. That's the basis of the calories in vs. calories out equation. However, the TLC diet isn't just about weight loss. To effectively lower cholesterol and reduce the risk of heart disease, certain foods must be eliminated or drastically reduced. The diet encourages nutrient-dense whole foods like fruits, vegetables, grains, legumes, nuts, and seeds, which are all naturally lower in calories and saturated fat.

Sustainable for Long-Term Health

The TLC diet was designed as a long-term solution to the widespread risk for heart disease. While followers might start to see results in a matter of months, they can drastically improve their cholesterol levels and heart disease markers if they stick with it for the long haul.

Cons

Might Be Outdated

One of the biggest critiques of the TLC diet is that it's outdated. Many of the studies on the TLC diet are from the early 2000s. There's concern that some of the suggestions of the TLC diet manual are unnecessary, such as reducing dietary cholesterol to 200 mg per day.

A 2020 report published in Circulation indicates that healthy dietary patterns can reduce the risk of heart disease more effectively than a specific target for dietary cholesterol. "A recommendation that gives a specific dietary cholesterol target within the context of food-based advice is challenging for clinicians and consumers to implement," the researchers concluded.7

Requires Diligent Tracking

The TLC diet has specific calorie and macronutrient requirements for its followers. People on this diet must diligently track their food intake to ensure that they meet these requirements.

Not Accommodating to Dietary Restrictions

For those with food allergies, adjusting the TLC diet requires some creativity. The manual doesn't offer advice for people who avoid certain foods that are recommended on this diet. With a few modifications, however, the TLC diet can still suit the needs of these individuals. Vegans or vegetarians, for example, can adopt a meatless TLC diet by swapping out lean meats for soy protein or legumes.

Is the TLC Diet a Healthy Choice for You?

The TLC diet isn't the only diet that claims to reduce cholesterol levels and the risk of heart disease. Many diets that encourage heart health tend to emphasize whole foods that are naturally lower in fat. They also tend to be restrictive. Similar heart-healthy diets include:

Whole foods diet: Like the TLC diet, the whole foods diet encourages unprocessed foods that are naturally lower in calories, saturated fat, salt, and sugar. This is typically regarded as a safe and nutritious diet.

Engine 2 diet: This restrictive diet eliminates animal products and vegetable oils. It's known to have heart health benefits and also aid in weight loss.

Mediterranean diet: Widely known for its heavy use of olive oil, the Mediterranean diet is also associated with a reduced risk of heart disease.10 It's also low in processed foods yet high in fiber. However, this diet may be higher in fat than the TLC diet. In terms of how the TLC diet compares to advice from health experts, there is certainly a lot of overlap. The U.S. Department of Agriculture's 2020–2025 Dietary Guidelines for Americans recommends a variety of nutrient-rich foods like fruits, vegetables, whole grains, lean protein sources, low-fat dairy products, and healthy fats for a well-balanced diet.11 While the USDA's guidelines are for the general public, the TLC diet is designed specifically with heart health in mind.

The TLC diet is especially low in saturated fat and dietary cholesterol compared to the USDA's recommendations. For adults, the USDA advises no more than 10% of total daily calories from saturated fat.11 The TLC diet is more strict, with a recommendation of fewer than 7% of calories from saturated fat.

Current federal guidelines indicate that dietary cholesterol consumption should be "as low as possible"11 without citing a specific number (previous editions of the guidelines have indicated no more than 300 mg). The TLC diet has a maximum dietary cholesterol intake of 200 mg. The USDA advises that the number of calories needed to maintain a healthy weight varies based on age, sex, and level of physical activity.11 Those following the TLC diet are also advised to keep track of their daily intake of both calories and macronutrients. Use this calculator to estimate a daily calorie target to help you stay on track with your goals.

Health Benefits

The TLC diet has been shown to reduce cholesterol, decrease the risk of heart disease, lower blood pressure, and more.12 It may also help stabilize blood sugar and reduce oxidative stress.13

This plan can also be an effective strategy for weight loss and weight maintenance.14 By consuming fewer calories, exercising regularly, and choosing foods that are low-fat, high-fiber, and nutrient-dense, followers can lose weight in a healthy and sustainable way. While the TLC diet is arguably a healthy choice, some aspects of the plan's guidelines may be out of date. For instance, a 2020 report published in Circulation indicates that healthy dietary patterns can reduce the risk of heart disease more effectively than a specific target for dietary cholesterol, hence why some experts say the TLC diet's limit on dietary cholesterol is unnecessary.

"A recommendation that gives a specific dietary cholesterol target within the context of food-based advice is challenging for clinicians and consumers to implement," the researchers concluded.

THE TLC DIET RECIPES

Grilled salmon with avocado salsa

Recipe for grilled salmon with avocado salsa, the fish is seasoned with coriander, cumin, paprika, onion powder and pepper, and topped with avocado salsa.

Ingredients

• 2 lbs salmon cut into 4 to 6 fillets

• 1 tbs olive oil

• 1 tsp salt

• 1 tsp ground coriander

• 1 tsp ground cumin

• 1 tsp paprika powder

• 1 tsp onion powder

• 1 tsp black pepper

Avocado salsa

• 1 avocado peeled, seeded and sliced

• 1 small red onion sliced

- 3 mild hot peppers seeded and deveined, diced or sliced

- Juice from 2 limes

- 3 tbs olive oil

- 2 tbs finely chopped cilantro

- Salt to taste

Instructions

1. Mix the salt, coriander, cumin, paprika, onion and black pepper together, rub the salmon fillets with olive oil and this seasoning mix, and refrigerate for at least 30 minutes.

2. Pre-heat the grill.

3. Combine the avocado, onion, hot peppers, cilantro, lime juice, olive oil and salt in a bowl and mix well, chill until ready to use.

4. Grill the salmon to desired doneness.

5. Serve the salmon topped with the avocado salsa, and with rice and patacones or thick green plantain chips on the side.

This exceptional lamb loin recipe from Chris Horridge features a wonderful combination of elements, with blushing lamb served on a bed of creamy Parmesan risotto and wilted spinach, finished off with roast shallots, wild mushrooms and olives.

Ingredients

• 2 lamb loins

• 1 tbsp of olive oil

• 10g of butter

• 2 garlic cloves, peeled and chopped

• 1 sprig of rosemary, leaves stripped and chopped

• Parmesan Risotto

• 20g of butter

• 20g of shallots, diced

• 100g of risotto rice

• 375ml of water

• 100g of Parmesan, grated

- 1 tbsp of truffle oil

- Salt

- black pepper

- Spinach

- 400g of spinach

- 10g of butter

- Roast Shallots

- 4 banana shallots, peeled

- olive oil

- Salt

- Wild mushrooms

- 50g of wild mushrooms

- 20g of butter

To plate

- 1 handful of micro parsley

- 10 black olives

Method

• Remove the meat from the fridge and leave to sit at room temperature for one hour. Melt the butter over a medium heat and sweat the shallots without browning for 2 minutes. Add the rice to the shallots and cook for a further 2 mintues

• Pour over half the water and bring to a simmer. Season with salt and pepper. Lower the heat and cook slowly for 14 minutes, adding the water gradually and seasoning as required

• Remove from the heat, add the parmesan cheese and truffle oil. Stir gently with a plastic spatula. Pour onto a tray and cover until required

• Heat the oven to 180°C/gas mark 4. Coat the shallots in a little olive oil and salt and roast in the oven for 45 minutes until tender. Remove from the oven and leave to cool before slicing in half length ways

• Heat the oven to 180°C/Gas mark 4 so that it is ready for the lamb. In an ovenproof frying pan, cook the lamb loins on a high heat in 1 tablespoon of oil, colouring them evenly all over

• Add a knob of butter and continue to cook until nicely caramelized, which should take approximately 3-4 minutes

• Season. Cook in the oven for 5 minutes. Add the garlic and rosemary and coat the lamb. Rest on a plate with all the roasting juices. Place the roasted shallots in the oven to gently warm through for a few minutes

• Sweat the spinach in the butter. Drain well, pressing it between two cloths to soak up the excess water

• Warm the risotto in a pan, adding a little water if needed, then cook until hot and has the consistency of rice pudding

• In a small pan, melt the butter on a medium to high heat. Once it begins to foam, add the wild mushrooms and saute until golden and remove from the heat. Slice the cheeks of flesh off the olives and add to the pan to warm through

• Spoon the risotto onto the plate and place a line of spinach on top. Slice the lamb and season each slice, then place on top of the spinach. Place the shallots, mushrooms and olives around, spoon over some pan juices. Finish with the micro-parsley

Coconut Yoghurt Chicken

This succulent coconut yoghurt chicken is incredibly easy and requires only a handful of ingredients. It's paleo, Whole30, keto and gluten-free friendly and can be served with a lovely salad, cauliflower rice or zucchini noodles.

Ingredients

• 150 g / 5 oz. coconut yoghurt, unsweetened (dairy-free)

• 3 heaped teaspoons mild curry powder

• 1 teaspoon salt

• 500 g / 1 lb chicken tenderloins (about 6 pieces, you can also use sliced chicken breast or chicken thighs)

• Cooking oil such as macadamia or coconut oil

To finish:

• 2 tablespoons desiccated coconut, toasted or raw (optional)

• Juice of 1/2 lime

• A small handful of fresh coriander and chopped spring onions/scallions (optional)

Instructions

• Combine coconut yoghurt, curry powder and salt in a bowl. Add the chicken pieces and coat well with the marinade. Transfer the chicken and any leftover sauce to an airtight container and allow to marinate overnight or for at least 2 hours.

• To cook the chicken, heat 2 tablespoons of coconut oil or macadamia oil in a large frying pan over medium-high heat. Once the pan is hot, add the chicken pieces (don't worry about brushing off the marinade) and cook for 5 minutes until golden brown on one side.

• Use a spatula and slide it under the chicken, making sure to scrape the cooked marinade with it and turn over the pieces. Cook for another 3-4 minutes on the other side. If the pan is small, you might need to do the chicken in batches.

• After 8-10 minutes of cooking, add the remaining marinade in the gaps between the chicken pieces and cook over high heat for about 30 seconds to a minute. The sauce will start to bubble and thicken, caramelising on the bottom. At this stage, remove from heat.

• Finish the chicken by drizzling the juice of half lime over the top and sprinkling with toasted coconut and some fresh coriander and spring onions.

The BEST oven baked sweet potato fries recipe - with a trick to make them SUPER CRISPY! Learn how to make crispy baked sweet potato fries, using just 3 ingredients.

Ingredients

• 5 medium Sweet potatoes (peeled and sliced into fries, about 1/2 inch wide, 1/4 inch thick, and as long as you'd like)

• 2 tablespoons Olive oil

• 1 1/2 teaspoons Arrowroot powder

• Sea salt (to taste)

Instructions

1. Soak the sweet potato fries in a bowl of water. Leave the fries to soak in the water for at least 60 minutes (you can leave them as long as overnight).

2. Preheat the oven to 400 degrees F. Line a large baking sheet with parchment paper or a silicone mat.

3. Remove the fries from the water and pat dry. Transfer them to a bowl, add the olive oil, and mix until completely coated.

4. Sprinkle the arrowroot powder over the fries and toss to coat, breaking up any clumps.

5. Spread the prepared sweet potato fries evenly on the prepared baking sheet. Try to ensure that the fries don't touch each other on the tray to ensure an even bake.

6. Bake the fries for 25-30 minutes, until they are browned and crisp.

Colorful Roasted Sheet-Pan Veggies

These easy roasted vegetables will give your plate a pop of color. Give the cubes of butternut squash a head start for 10 minutes to soften in the oven before adding in the other veggies. The broccoli, peppers and onion are naturally more tender than the butternut squash and cook more quickly. That way everything ends up finishing at the same time.

Ingredients

3 cups cubed butternut squash (1-inch)

3 tablespoons extra-virgin olive oil, divided

4 cups broccoli florets

2 red bell peppers, cut into squares

1 large red onion, cut into bite-size chunks

2 teaspoons Italian seasoning or herbes de Provence

1 teaspoon coarse kosher salt

¼ teaspoon pepper

1 tablespoon best-quality balsamic vinegar

Directions

• Preheat oven to 425 degrees F.

• Toss squash and 1 tablespoon oil in a large bowl. Spread out on a baking sheet. Roast for 10 minutes.

• Meanwhile, toss broccoli, bell peppers, onion, Italian seasoning (or herbes de Provence), salt and pepper in the bowl with the remaining 2 tablespoons olive oil until the vegetables are evenly coated.

• Add the squash to the vegetables in the bowl. Toss to combine. Spread the vegetables out on 2 baking sheets, dividing evenly. Roast, stirring once or twice, until the vegetables are tender and browned in spots, 17 to 20 minutes. Drizzle with vinegar.

Here we marinate tofu cubes in soy sauce and lime juice with a touch of toasted sesame oil, then roast them-- perfect tofu every time.

Ingredients

2 (14 ounce) packages extra-firm, water-packed tofu, drained

⅔ cup reduced-sodium soy sauce

⅔ cup lime juice

6 tablespoons toasted sesame oil

Instructions

• Pat tofu dry and cut into 1/2- to 3/4-inch cubes. Combine soy sauce, lime juice and oil in a medium bowl or large sealable plastic bag. Add the tofu; gently toss to combine. Marinate in the refrigerator for 1 hour or up to 4 hours, gently stirring once or twice.

• Preheat oven to 450 degrees F.

• Remove the tofu from the marinade with a slotted spoon (discard marinade). Spread out on 2 large baking sheets, making sure the pieces are not touching. Roast, gently turning halfway through, until golden brown, about 20 minutes.

Shredded Chicken Master Recipe

This easy slow-cooker method preps chicken for a multitude of recipes. Bonus: Rich-tasting chicken stock to keep on hand in your freezer as well.

Ingredients

4 1/2 to 5 pounds chicken thighs, skinned

4 fresh thyme sprigs

4 fresh parsley stems

2 bay leaves

2 cloves garlic, halved

½ teaspoon whole black peppercorns

1 (32 ounce) carton reduced-sodium chicken broth

Instructions

Place chicken thighs in a 4- to 5-quart slow cooker. For the bouquet garni, place thyme sprigs, parsley stems, bay leaves, garlic, and peppercorns in the center of a double-thick 8-inch square of 100%-cotton cheesecloth. Gather corners together and tie closed with 100%-cotton kitchen string. Add bouquet garni to slow cooker. Pour broth over all in cooker.

Cover and cook on low-heat setting for 7 to 8 hours or on high-heat setting for 3 1/2 to 4 hours. Remove bouquet garni and discard.

Using a slotted spoon, transfer chicken to a large bowl, reserving cooking liquid. When chicken is cool enough to handle, remove meat from bones. Using two forks, shred meat. Add enough of the cooking liquid to moisten meat. Strain and reserve cooking liquid to use for chicken stock.

Muffin-Tin Quiches with Smoked Cheddar & Potato

Potatoes, cheese and greens make this mini quiche recipe delicious and satisfying. Bake up a batch over the weekend and you'll have breakfast available in a hurry for the rest of the week.

Ingredients

2 tablespoons extra-virgin olive oil

1 ½ cups finely diced red-skinned potatoes

1 cup diced red onion

¾ teaspoon salt, divided

8 large eggs

1 cup shredded smoked Cheddar cheese

½ cup low-fat milk

½ teaspoon ground black pepper

1 ½ cups chopped fresh spinach

Instructions

Preheat oven to 325 degrees F. Coat a 12-cup muffin tin with cooking spray.

Heat oil in a large skillet over medium heat. Add potatoes, onion and 1/4 teaspoon salt and cook, stirring, until the potatoes are just cooked through, about 5 minutes. Remove from heat and let cool 5 minutes.

Whisk eggs, cheese, milk, pepper and the remaining 1/2 teaspoon salt in a large bowl. Stir in spinach and the potato mixture. Divide the ⍰uiche mixture among the prepared muffin cups.

Bake until firm to the touch, about 25 minutes. Let stand 5 minutes before removing from the tin.

Chicken Sausage and Peppers

Colorful peppers and tomatoes and sweet onion make this sausage dinner pop with fresh flavor. Roasting instead of sautéing makes this even easier for a busy weeknight.

Ingredients

Nonstick cooking spray

4 medium red, yellow, orange, and/or green sweet peppers, cut into 1-inch pieces

1 large sweet onion, cut into thin wedges

2 cups grape tomatoes

1 tablespoon olive oil

1 tablespoon balsamic vinegar

1 (12 ounce) package Italian-flavor cooked chicken sausage, such as Al Fresco brand, bias-sliced into thirds

1 tablespoon snipped fresh oregano

8 Toasted baguette slices

Instructions

Preheat oven to 425 degrees F. Coat a 15x10-inch baking pan with cooking spray. In the prepared pan combine peppers, onion, and tomatoes. Drizzle with oil and vinegar; toss gently to coat. Roast 30 minutes.

Push vegetables to one side, exposing about one-fourth of the pan. Place sausage in pan. Roast 10 to 15 minutes more or until vegetables are tender and sausage is heated through. Sprinkle with oregano. If desired, serve with toasted baguette slices.

Here's the only recipe you need to make perfect brown rice every time! This healthy whole grain is great on its own as a side dish, or use it in your favorite recipes calling for cooked brown rice.

Ingredients

2 ½ cups water or broth

1 cup brown rice

Instruction

Combine water (or broth) and rice in a medium saucepan. Bring to a boil. Reduce heat to low, cover and simmer until tender and most of the liquid has been absorbed, 40 to 50 minutes. Let stand 5 minutes, then fluff with a fork.

Cherry-Chocolate Chip Granola Bars

Skip the granola bar options at the grocery store--they're easy to make at home! You can vary the add-ins to your taste, swapping 2 cups of any combination of small (or chopped) dried fruit, nuts and/or seeds for the chocolate, cherries and coconut in this version. We tested several sticky sweeteners, including maple syrup and honey, but found brown rice syrup held the bars together the best.

Ingredients

3 cups old-fashioned rolled oats

1 cup crispy brown rice cereal

1 cup chopped dried cherries (1/4 inch)

⅓ cup unsalted almonds, toasted and chopped

⅓ cup mini chocolate chips

⅓ cup unsweetened shredded coconut

¼ teaspoon salt

⅔ cup brown rice syrup or light corn syrup

½ cup almond butter

1 teaspoon vanilla extract

Instruction

Preheat oven to 325 degrees F. Line a 9-by-13-inch baking pan with parchment paper, leaving extra parchment hanging over two sides. Lightly coat the parchment with cooking spray.

Combine oats, rice cereal, cherries, almonds, chocolate chips, coconut and salt in a large mixing bowl.

Combine rice syrup (or corn syrup), almond butter and vanilla extract in a microwave-safe bowl. Microwave for 30 seconds (or heat in a saucepan over medium heat for 1 minute). Add to the dry ingredients and stir until evenly combined. Transfer to the prepared pan and firmly press into the pan with the back of a spatula.

For chewier bars, bake until barely starting to color around the edge and still soft in the middle, 20 to 25 minutes. For crunchier bars, bake until golden brown around the edge and somewhat firm in the middle, 30 to 35 minutes. (Both will still be soft when warm and firm up as they cool.)

Let cool in the pan for 10 minutes, then using the parchment to help you, lift out of the pan onto a cutting board (it will still be soft). Cut into 24 bars, then let cool completely without separating the bars, about 30 minutes more. Once cool, separate into bars.

Slow-Cooker Chicken Noodle Soup Meal-Prep Freezer Pack

Not only does this chicken noodle soup recipe utilize the crock pot for a set-it-and-forget-it easy dinner, you can also prep all the ingredients ahead of time and store them away in the freezer to pull out on a day where you forgot to plan dinner. That's a meal-prep win! Just make sure you thaw the food before adding it to the slow cooker-- otherwise it will remain at an unsafe temperature for too long.

Ingredients

8 ounces whole-wheat egg noodles or other whole-wheat noodles

3 pounds bone-in chicken breast, skin removed

2 cups chopped onion

1 cup chopped carrot

1 cup chopped celery

2 sprigs thyme

8 cups low-sodium chicken broth

2 teaspoons kosher salt

2 cups frozen peas

¼ cup chopped fresh dill, plus more for garnish

2 tablespoons lemon juice

Instructions

Cook noodles according to package directions. Drain and rinse with cold water to cool.

Meanwhile, place chicken, onion, carrot, celery and thyme in a sealable gallon-size freezer bag. Place the cooled noodles in a separate sealable gallon-size freezer bag. Freeze both bags until ready to use. Let the bags defrost in your refrigerator for 1 day before cooking (see Tip).

Combine the chicken mixture, broth and salt in a 6-quart slow cooker (reserve the noodles). Cook on High for 4 hours or Low for 8 hours. Add peas during the last 10 minutes of cooking.

Transfer the chicken to a clean cutting board. When the chicken is cool enough to handle, remove the meat from the bones and shred into bite-size pieces. Stir the chicken into the soup along with the noodles, dill and lemon juice. Garnish with more dill, if desired.

Avocado Hummus

This vibrant green hummus recipe couldn't be easier--just toss a few ingredients in the food processor and whir away! Aquafaba (the liquid from a can of chickpeas) and avocado make this healthy dip extra smooth and creamy. Serve with veggie chips, pita chips or crudités.

Ingredients

   1 (15 ounce) can no-salt-added chickpeas

   1 ripe avocado, halved and pitted

   1 cup fresh cilantro leaves

   ¼ cup tahini

   ¼ cup extra-virgin olive oil

   ¼ cup lemon juice

   1 clove garlic

   1 teaspoon ground cumin

   ½ teaspoon salt

Instruction

Drain chickpeas, reserving 2 tablespoons of the liquid. Transfer the chickpeas and the reserved liquid to a food processor. Add avocado, cilantro, tahini, oil, lemon juice, garlic, cumin and salt. Puree until very smooth. Serve with veggie chips, pita chips or crudités.

Sheet-Pan Roasted Root Vegetables

One pan is all you need for a heaping pile of nutritious, tender and colorful root vegetables. Whip up this large-batch recipe at the beginning of the week to use in easy, healthy dinners all week long.

Ingredients

2 large carrots

2 medium parsnips, peeled

2 medium beets, peeled

1 medium red onion

1 medium sweet potato

3 tablespoons extra-virgin olive oil

1 ½ tablespoons apple cider vinegar or balsamic vinegar

1 tablespoon fresh herbs, such as thyme, rosemary or sage

½ teaspoon kosher salt

½ teaspoon ground pepper

Instructions

Position racks in upper and lower thirds of oven; preheat to 425 degrees F. Line 2 large baking sheets with parchment paper.

Cut carrots and parsnips into 1/2-inch-thick slices on a diagonal, then cut into half moons. Cut beets and onion into 1/2-inch-thick wedges. Cut sweet potato into 3/4-inch cubes. You should have about 12 cups raw vegetables.

Toss the vegetables with oil, vinegar, herbs, salt and pepper in a large bowl until well coated. Divide between the prepared baking sheets, spreading into a single layer.

Roast the vegetables, rotating the pans top to bottom halfway through, until fork-tender, 30 to 40 minutes.

Vegan Freezer Breakfast Burritos

Having a stash of flavorful bean burritos in your freezer means you'll always have a satisfying plant-based meal ready for a grab-and-go breakfast on a busy morning or to take to the campsite for an easy campfire meal. Our vegan breakfast filling--made with tofu and prepared to mimic scrambled eggs--is tossed with beans, veggies and salsa for a delicious and ultra-satisfying meal.

Ingredients

2 tablespoons avocado oil, divided

1 (14 ounce) package extra-firm water-packed tofu, drained and crumbled

2 teaspoons chili powder

1 teaspoon ground cumin

¼ teaspoon salt

1 (15 ounce) can reduced-sodium black beans, rinsed

1 cup frozen corn, thawed

4 scallions, sliced

½ cup prepared fresh salsa

¼ cup chopped fresh cilantro

6 (8 inch) whole-wheat tortillas or wraps

Instruction

Heat 1 tablespoon oil in a large nonstick skillet over medium heat. Add tofu, chili powder, cumin and salt; cook, stirring, until the tofu is nicely browned, 10 to 12 minutes. Transfer to a bowl.

Add the remaining 1 tablespoon oil to the pan. Add beans, corn and scallions and cook, stirring, until the scallions have softened, about 3 minutes. Return the tofu to the pan. Add salsa and cilantro; cook, stirring, until heated through, about 2 minutes more.

If serving immediately, warm tortillas (or wraps; see Tip), but if freezing do not warm them. Divide the bean mixture among the tortillas, spreading evenly over the bottom third of each tortilla. Roll snugly, tucking in the ends as you go. Serve immediately or wrap each burrito in foil and freeze for up to 3 months.

To heat in the microwave: Remove foil, cover with a paper towel and microwave on High until hot, 1 1/2 to 2 minutes.

To heat over a campfire: Place foil-wrapped burrito on a cooking grate over a medium to medium-hot fire. Cook, turning once or twice, until steaming hot throughout, 5 to 10 minutes if partially thawed, up to 15 minutes if frozen.

The quick 10-minute Spicy Cabbage Slaw serves as the low-carb base in this veggie-packed lunch recipe. Topped with high-protein edamame and shrimp, this satisfying lunch will help you power through the afternoon.

Ingredients

1 recipe Spicy Cabbage Slaw (see associated recipe)

2 cups frozen shelled edamame, thawed

1 medium avocado, diced

½ medium lime, juiced

12 ounces peeled cooked shrimp

Instructions

Prepare Spicy Cabbage Slaw. Add edamame; toss and set aside.

Toss avocado with lime juice in a small bowl.

Divide the slaw mixture among 4 containers. Top each with 1/4 of the shrimp (about 3 ounces) and 1/4 of the avocado. Cover and refrigerate until ready to eat.

Meal-Prep Cilantro-Lime Chicken Bowls

Prep all four servings of this easy recipe at once for ready-to-eat dinners or packable lunches for the rest of the week. If you don't like a lot of heat, try using mild chili powder, and leave out the jalapeño from the rice.

Ingredients

1 pound boneless, skinless chicken breasts, cut into 1-inch pieces

¾ teaspoon salt, divided

½ teaspoon chipotle chile powder or mild chili powder

¼ teaspoon ground pepper

3 tablespoons extra-virgin olive oil, divided

¼ cup chopped fresh cilantro

1 medium red onion, sliced

1 red bell pepper, sliced

1 green bell pepper, sliced

2 cups cooked brown rice

1 medium tomato, chopped

1 tablespoon chopped jalapeño pepper (Optional)

1 (15 ounce) can reduced-sodium black beans, rinsed

½ cup crumbled ueso fresco (2 1/2 ounces)

1 lime, cut into 4 wedges

Instructions

Toss chicken with 1/4 teaspoon salt, chipotle (or chili) powder and pepper in a medium bowl. Heat 2 tablespoons oil in a large skillet over medium-high heat. Add the chicken and cook, stirring occasionally, until browned and cooked through, 6 to 8 minutes. Transfer the chicken to a clean bowl and let cool slightly. Toss with cilantro and set aside.

Meanwhile, add the remaining 1 tablespoon oil to the pan. Add onion, red pepper, green pepper and 1/4 teaspoon salt. Cook over medium heat, stirring occasionally, until the vegetables have softened and are beginning to brown, 6 to 8 minutes. Reduce heat if vegetables are getting too dark.

Combine rice, tomato, jalapeño, if using, and the remaining 1/4 teaspoon salt in a medium bowl.

To assemble: Divide equal portions of black beans, the chicken mixture, bell pepper mixture and rice mixture among 4 microwave-safe containers. Top each with queso fresco and a lime wedge. Refrigerate until ready to use (up to 4 days).

To reheat, remove the lime wedge. Microwave each container on High for 1 to 2 minutes, or until heated through. Squeeze the lime wedge over the top.

Roasted Salmon Rice Bowl with Beets & Brussels

Roasting vegetables and salmon together on one sheet pan while the rice cooks makes an easy, satisfying meal packed with protein, whole grains and veggies. To ensure that you're getting 100 percent whole grains, look for a wild rice blend that consists of wild and brown rice.

Ingredients

1 cup wild rice blend

2 medium golden beets, peeled and cut into 1/2-inch wedges

8 ounces Brussels sprouts, trimmed and halved

3 tablespoons extra-virgin olive oil, divided

¾ teaspoon salt, divided

¾ teaspoon ground pepper, divided

1 lemon

1 pound wild-caught salmon fillet, cut into 4 portions

2 rosemary sprigs, cut in half

2 tablespoons chopped fresh herbs, such as thyme, basil or rosemary

1 clove garlic, minced

1 tablespoon chopped pistachios

Instructions

Preheat oven to 425 degrees F.

Cook rice blend according to package directions.

Meanwhile, toss beets and Brussels sprouts with 1 tablespoon oil and 1/4 teaspoon each salt and pepper in a medium bowl. After the rice has cooked for 10 minutes, spread the vegetables on a large rimmed baking sheet and roast until just beginning to brown and soften, about 15 minutes.

Cut lemon in half crosswise. Cut half the lemon into 4 slices (reserve the other lemon half). Push the beets and Brussels sprouts to one side of the baking sheet and place salmon on the empty half. Sprinkle the salmon with 1/4 teaspoon each salt and pepper and top each piece of salmon with a rosemary sprig and a lemon slice. Continue roasting until the vegetables have softened and the salmon is opaque in the center, 9 to 11 minutes more.

Meanwhile, squeeze the juice from the remaining lemon half into a small bowl. Whisk in the remaining 2 tablespoons oil, herbs, garlic and the remaining 1/4 teaspoon each salt and pepper.

Divide the rice among 4 bowls. Discard the lemon slices and rosemary sprig. Arrange the salmon and vegetables on top of the rice. Drizzle each serving with about 1 tablespoon lemon juice mixture and sprinkle with pistachios.

Blueberry-Banana Overnight Oats

Blueberries, sweet banana and creamy coconut milk combine to turn everyday oatmeal into the best vegan overnight oats! Make up to 4 jars at once to keep in the fridge for quick grab-and-go breakfasts throughout the week.

Ingredients

½ cup unsweetened coconut milk beverage

½ cup old-fashioned oats (see Tip)

½ tablespoon chia seeds (Optional)

½ banana, mashed

1 teaspoon maple syrup

Pinch of salt

½ cup fresh blueberries

1 tablespoon unsweetened flaked coconut (Optional)

Instruction

Combine coconut milk, oats, chia seeds (if using), banana, maple syrup and salt in a pint-sized jar and stir. Top with blueberries and coconut, if desired. Cover and refrigerate overnight.

Save time and maximize your efforts by mixing up two separate chicken marinades and cooking multiple recipes at once. This simple but flavorful meal-prep chicken dinner idea lets you cook ahead and not be bored with your choices by mid-week. Both recipes are roasted together on a baking sheet; a foil barrier keeps them separate. Make this base chicken recipe and use it to create the Meal-Prep Chili-Lime Chicken Bowls & Meal-Prep Curried Chicken Bowls (see associated recipes) for lunch or dinner this week.

Ingredients

Curried Chicken

    ¾ cup low-fat plain yogurt

    ⅓ cup grated onion

    2 tablespoons mild curry powder

    1 ½ tablespoons lemon juice

    1 tablespoon extra-virgin olive oil

    ½ teaspoon salt

¼ teaspoon cayenne pepper (optional)

1 pound boneless, skinless chicken breast, cut into 1-inch pieces

Chili-Lime Chicken

2 tablespoons extra-virgin olive oil

1 tablespoon chili powder

1 teaspoon lime zest

1 ½ tablespoons lime juice

2 cloves garlic, grated

1 teaspoon ground cumin

½ teaspoon salt

1 pound boneless, skinless chicken breast, cut into 1-inch pieces

Instructions

To prepare Curried Chicken: Stir yogurt, onion, curry powder, lemon juice, oil, salt and cayenne, if using, together in a medium bowl. Add chicken and toss to coat.

Cover and marinate in the refrigerator for at least 2 hours or overnight.

To prepare Chili-Lime Chicken: Stir oil, chili powder, lime zest and juice, garlic, cumin and salt together in a medium bowl. Add chicken and toss to coat. Cover and marinate in the refrigerator for at least 2 hours or overnight.

Preheat oven to 400 degrees F. Line a rimmed baking sheet with foil and create a foil barrier to divide the baking sheet in half.

Place the Curried Chicken, in a single layer, on one side of the foil and the Chili-Lime Chicken, in a single layer, on the other side of the foil. Roast until the chicken is cooked through, 15 to 18 minutes.

Apple Spice Muffins

Think of crème fraîche as sour cream's richer, thicker, less-sour sibling. In this healthy muffin recipe, it's the secret ingredient that gives these muffins a light texture and rich flavor. The batter is made with extra spices and tons of sweet fruit, which means you won't notice the minimal amount of white sugar.

Ingredients

Muffin Batter

1 ¾ cups white whole-wheat flour

2 teaspoons baking powder

2 teaspoons ground cinnamon

1 teaspoon ground ginger

½ teaspoon baking soda

½ teaspoon kosher salt

¼ teaspoon ground cloves

⅓ cup granulated sugar

8 tablespoons unsalted butter (1 stick), melted and at room temperature

½ cup crème fraîche, at room temperature

½ cup reduced-fat milk, at room temperature

2 large eggs

1 tablespoon vanilla extract

¾ cup dried cranberries or raisins, divided

3 ½ cups finely chopped peeled Granny Smith apples (2-3 large)

1 cup rolled oats

Crumb Topping

¾ cup rolled oats

½ cup white whole-wheat flour

1 teaspoon ground cinnamon

¼ teaspoon kosher salt

4 tablespoons unsalted butter (1/2 stick), melted

3 tablespoons honey

2 teaspoons vanilla extract

Instructions

Position racks in upper and lower thirds of oven; preheat to 350 degrees F. Line 20 muffin cups with paper liners.

To prepare batter: Sift 1 3/4 cups flour, baking powder, 2 teaspoons cinnamon, ginger, baking soda, 1/2 teaspoon salt and cloves into a mixing bowl. Add sugar and 8 tablespoons butter and stir to combine. Add crème fraîche, milk, eggs and 1 tablespoon vanilla; beat on low speed for 10 to 15 seconds. Increase speed to medium-high and beat until light and fluffy, about 20 seconds.

Chop about half the cranberries (or raisins) into small pieces. Fold all the cranberries (or raisins), apples and 1 cup oats into the batter. Divide the batter among the prepared muffin cups.

To prepare topping: Mix oats, flour, cinnamon and salt in a medium bowl. Whisk butter, honey and vanilla in a small bowl; drizzle on top of the oat mixture and mix until well incorporated. Top each muffin with some of the crumb topping.

Bake on the upper and lower racks, rotating top to bottom halfway through, until lightly golden and firm to the touch, 30 to 35 minutes. Let cool in the tins on a wire rack for at least 30 minutes before serving.

Creamy Blueberry-Pecan Overnight Oatmeal

These overnight oats with Greek yogurt, blueberries and pecans are an easy, on-the-go-breakfast. If desired, reheat the oatmeal before adding the toppings.

Ingredients

½ cup old-fashioned rolled oats

½ cup water

Pinch of salt

½ cup blueberries, fresh or frozen, thawed

2 tablespoons nonfat plain Greek yogurt

1 tablespoon toasted chopped pecans

2 teaspoons pure maple syrup

Instructions

Combine oats, water and salt in a jar or bowl. Cover and refrigerate overnight. In the morning, heat if desired, and top with blueberries, yogurt, pecans and syrup.

This easy-to-make and meal-prep burrito bowl is even better than takeout! You'll never miss the carbs in this protein-packed, super-flavorful meal that replaces the cilantro-lime rice with cauliflower rice. We love this with chicken but it would be just as delicious with shrimp.

Ingredients

4 cups cauliflower florets

3 tablespoons extra-virgin olive oil, divided

½ teaspoon salt, divided

1 pound skinless, boneless chicken breasts

1 tablespoon finely chopped chipotle peppers in adobo sauce

½ teaspoon garlic powder

½ teaspoon ground cumin

2 cups shredded romaine lettuce

1 cup canned pinto beans, rinsed

1 ripe avocado, diced

¼ cup pico de gallo or fresh salsa

¼ cup shredded Cheddar or Monterey Jack cheese

Lime wedges for serving

Instructions

Pulse cauliflower in a food processor until chopped into rice-size pieces. Heat 2 tablespoons oil in a large skillet over medium-high heat. Add the cauliflower and 1/4 teaspoon salt. Cook, stirring occasionally, until the cauliflower is softened, about 5 minutes. Cover and keep warm.

Position a rack in upper third of oven; preheat broiler to high. Coat a large rimmed baking sheet with cooking spray.

Season chicken with the remaining 1/4 teaspoon salt. Place on the prepared baking sheet and broil for 9 minutes.

Meanwhile, combine the remaining 1 tablespoon oil, chipotles, garlic powder and cumin in a small bowl.

Turn the chicken over, brush with the chipotle glaze and continue broiling until an instant-read thermometer inserted in the thickest part registers 165 degrees F, 8 to 10 minutes more. Transfer to a clean cutting board and chop into bite-size pieces.

Assemble each bowl with 1/2 cup each cauliflower rice, chicken and lettuce, 1/4 cup beans, 1/4 avocado and 1 tablespoon each pico de gallo (or salsa) and cheese. Serve with a lime wedge.

Fruit & Nuts Snack Mix

Whip up a big batch of this sweet and salty mix for on-the-go fuel or to have on hand for after-school snacks.

Ingredients

  1 cup lightly salted peanuts

  1 cup yogurt-covered raisins

  1 cup mini pretzels

  1 cup sweetened dried cranberries

Instructions

Combine peanuts, raisins, pretzels and cranberries in a large bowl.

Making a big batch of eggs has never been easier with this one-pan oven-baked eggs recipe. Whether you are making brunch for a crowd or just want to meal-prep healthy breakfasts for the week, you'll have 12 servings ready in just 45 minutes.

Ingredients

18 large eggs

¼ cup reduced-fat milk

1 ½ teaspoons smoked paprika

1 teaspoon salt

1 teaspoon ground pepper

1 teaspoon onion powder

1 (10 ounce) package frozen chopped spinach, thawed and squeezed dry

1 cup shredded sharp Cheddar cheese

½ cup diced ham

Instructions

Preheat oven to 300 degrees F. Generously coat a large rimmed baking sheet with cooking spray.

Whisk eggs, milk, smoked paprika, salt, pepper and onion powder together in a large bowl. Pour onto the prepared baking sheet and sprinkle with spinach, Cheddar and ham. Bake until just set, 20 to 25 minutes, rotating the pan from back to front halfway through baking to ensure even cooking. Cut into 12 squares and serve.

Citrus Lime Tofu Salad

This veggie-packed salad has plenty of protein and fiber, so you'll feel full and satisfied. Prep the ingredients ahead of time for an easy vegan lunch idea to pack for work.

Ingredients

2 cups mixed greens

1 cup roasted vegetables, chopped if desired (see associated recipes)

1 cup roasted tofu (see associated recipes)

1 tablespoon pumpkin seeds

2 tablespoons Citrus-Lime Vinaigrette (see associated recipes)

Instructions

Arrange greens, veggies, tofu and pumpkin seeds in a 4-cup sealable container or bowl. Drizzle vinaigrette over the salad just before serving

Chicken Curry Cup of Noodles

Make your own cup of instant soup at home with this chicken curry zoodle (spiralized zucchini noodles) recipe. Pack several jars at once to take to work for easy lunches throughout the week.

Ingredients

3 teaspoons reduced-sodium chicken bouillon paste, divided

6 teaspoons red curry paste, divided

6 tablespoons coconut milk, divided

1 ½ cups frozen stir-fry vegetable mix, divided

9 ounces chopped cooked boneless, skinless chicken breast, divided

1 ½ cups spiralized zucchini noodles, divided

3 teaspoons chopped cilantro, divided

3 cups very hot water, divided

Instructions

Add 1 teaspoon bouillon paste, 2 teaspoons curry paste and 2 tablespoons coconut milk to each of three 1 1/2-pint canning jars. Layer 1/2 cup vegetables, 3 ounces chicken and 1/2 cup noodles in each jar. Top each with 1 teaspoon cilantro. Cover and refrigerate for up to 3 days.

To prepare one jar of noodles: Add 1 cup very hot water to a jar. Cover and shake to combine. Uncover and microwave on High in 1-minute increments until steaming hot, 2 to 3 minutes total. Let stand 5 minutes. Stir before eating.

Classic Cobb Mason Jar Salad

Pack classic Cobb salad upside down in a mason jar for a healthy lunch that won't get soggy while sitting in the fridge all morning. Or pack it up the night before for an easy grab-and-go lunch in the morning.

Ingredients

2 tablespoons Creamy Blue Cheese Dressing (see associated recipe)

2 tablespoons chopped cucumber

2 tablespoons chopped tomato

2 tablespoons diced red onion

1 ounce chopped low- or reduced-sodium deli ham

1 ounce chopped low- or reduced-sodium deli turkey

1 hard-boiled egg, diced

1 slice crisply cooked bacon, crumbled

½ avocado, cubed

1 teaspoon lime juice

1 tablespoon crumbled blue cheese

1 ½ cups chopped romaine lettuce

Instructions

Add blue cheese dressing to a quart-size mason jar. Top with cucumber, tomato and onion. Layer in ham, turkey, egg and bacon. Gently toss avocado with lime juice in a small bowl, then add to the jar. Top the salad with blue cheese. Fill the remaining space in the jar with lettuce. Put the lid on the jar and refrigerate.

When ready to serve, shake the salad from the jar into a bowl.

Quinoa & Chia Oatmeal Mix

Make your own hot cereal mix with this healthy recipe. Keep it on hand and just cook up the amount you need when you're ready for a hot breakfast. One serving of the warm cereal contains 6 grams of fiber--almost a quarter of your daily quota-which helps stave off hunger throughout the morning.

Ingredients

2 cups old-fashioned rolled oats

1 cup rolled wheat and/or barley flakes (see Tip)

1 cup quinoa

1 cup dried fruit, such as raisins, cranberries and/or chopped apricots

½ cup chia and/or hemp seeds

1 teaspoon ground cinnamon

¾ teaspoon salt

Instructions

To make the hot cereal dry mix: Combine oats, wheat and/or barley flakes, Quinoa, dried fruit, seeds, cinnamon and salt in an airtight container.

To make 1 serving of hot cereal: Combine 1/3 cup Quinoa & Chia Oatmeal Mix with 1 1/4 cups water (or milk) in a small saucepan. Bring to a boil. Reduce heat, partially cover and simmer, stirring occasionally, until thickened, 12 to 15 minutes. Let stand, covered, for 5 minutes. Stir in a sweetener of your choice and top with nuts and/or more dried fruit, if desired. Makes 1 cup.

Freezer Bean & Cheese Burritos

This copycat version of store-bought frozen burritos is perfect for meal prepping. Make a big batch to store in the freezer for healthy packable lunches or a quick campsite meal.

Ingredients

1 ½ cups chopped grape tomatoes

4 scallions, chopped

¼ cup chopped pickled jalapeño peppers

2 tablespoons chopped fresh cilantro

2 (15 ounce) cans low-sodium pinto beans, rinsed

4 teaspoons chili powder

1 teaspoon ground cumin

2 cups shredded sharp Cheddar cheese

8 8-inch whole-wheat tortillas, at room temperature

Instructions

Combine tomatoes, scallions, jalapeños and cilantro in a medium bowl.

Mash beans with chili powder and cumin in a large bowl with a fork or potato masher until almost smooth. Add cheese and the tomato mixture and stir until combined. Spread about 1/2 cup of the filling mixture on the bottom third of each tortilla. Roll snugly, tucking in the ends as you go. Wrap each burrito in heavy-duty foil. Freeze for up to 3 months.

To heat in the microwave: Unwrap a burrito and place on a microwave-safe plate. Cover with a paper towel and microwave on High until steaming hot throughout, 1 1/2 to 2 1/2 minutes.

To heat over a campfire: Place foil-wrapped burrito on a cooking grate over a medium to medium-hot fire. Cook, turning once or twice, until steaming hot throughout, 5 to 10 minutes if partially thawed, up to 15 minutes if frozen.

Shredded Turkey & Pinto Bean Burritos

We created this with leftover turkey in mind. Leftover or rotisserie chicken can also be used. Make it a Meal: Serve with guacamole and chopped jalapeño peppers and/or hot sauce--and a cold cerveza.

Ingredients

1 tablespoon canola oil

1 medium onion, halved and sliced

2 cloves garlic, minced

1 tablespoon ground cumin

1 teaspoon chile powder

1 15-ounce can diced tomatoes with green chiles

2 tablespoons lime juice

4 cups shredded cooked turkey or chicken

1 15-ounce can pinto beans, rinsed

6 10-inch whole-wheat flour tortillas or wraps, warmed (see Tip)

¾ cup grated Monterey or pepper Jack cheese

2 cups shredded green cabbage

Instructions

Heat oil in a large saucepan over medium heat. Add onion and cook, stirring, until softened, about 2 minutes. Stir in garlic, cumin and chile powder and cook for 30 seconds. Add tomatoes and lime juice; bring to a boil. Reduce heat to a simmer and cook until the onions are very soft, 16 to 20 minutes. Stir in turkey (or chicken) and beans and continue cooking until the mixture is heated through, 3 to 5 minutes more.

Divide the turkey-bean mixture among tortillas (or wraps). Top each with cheese and cabbage, roll into burritos and serve.

Cola Chicken

Chicken that's easy to make and low calorie.

Ingredients

   3 chicken breasts

   1 can (12 oz) diet cola

   1 cup ketchup

Directions

Put chicken in a non-stick skillet.

Pour ketchup and diet cola (any kind) over the top.

Bring to a boil. Cover, reduce heat cook for 45 minutes.

Uncover, turn up the heat and continue to cook until the sauce becomes thick and adheres to the chicken. Be sure to watch it during this last step.

Sausage and Spinach Crustless Quiche is an easy low carb (keto) breakfast or brunch recipe loaded with sausage, cheese, and spinach.

Ingredients

1 pound Ground breakfast sausage

8 ounces Cream cheese, cubed

6 Eggs

1 cup Heavy Cream

8 ounces Cheddar cheese, shredded

5 ounces Fresh baby spinach

Instructions

Preheat oven to 375 degrees F.

In a skillet over medium high heat brown the ground breakfast sausage until it is almost cooked through. Drain excess grease and return to the skillet.

Add cream cheese and stir together with sausage cooking until the sausage finishes cooking and the cream cheese is fully melted.

Place baby spinach in a microwave-safe bowl and add 2 tablespoons of water. Microwave for 2-3 minutes until spinach is lightly steamed and tender.

In a bowl add eggs and 1 cup of heavy cream. Whisk together. Spoon the sausage cream cheese mixture into a greased 11x7 inch casserole dish.Add spinach on top of the sausage and sprinkle the shredded cheddar cheese over everything.

 Pour the egg mixture over the sausage and spinach and use a spoon to move things around just a big to let the eggs get down into the mixture.

Place in the oven and bake for 35-40 minutes or until you can jiggle the pan and the quiche doesn't shake in the center.

Remove and let cool for about 5 minutes before cutting and serving.

Cashew Chicken Lettuce Wraps

Cashew Chicken Lettuce Wraps for dinner tonight! A easy and delicious recipe that ⍰uickly whips together in under 30 minutes.

Ingredients

1 pound ground chicken

3 cloves garlic, minced

3 Tablespoons chili paste

2 Tablespoon rice vinegar (may omit if you don't have it on hand)

1/3 cup coconut aminos

2 Tablespoon erythritol (or sweetener of your choice)

1/2 teaspoon red pepper flakes (optional for extra heat)

1/4 teaspoon ground ginger (freshly minced gingers work great as well)

1/4 teaspoon black pepper

1/4 teaspoon sea salt + more to taste

1 cup cashews

1 head lettuce

Instructions

In a large skillet, cook ground chicken and garlic over medium-high heat. Cook until garlic is tender and chicken is cooked through.

Turn heat down to medium-low. Stir in chili paste, vinegar, coconut aminos, erythritol, red pepper flakes, ground ginger, black pepper, salt and cashews. Cook for another 6-8 minutes, or until sauce is combined and cashews turn color and are slightly tender but still a bit of a crunch in them.

Spoon filling into lettuce, add additional coconut aminos and red pepper flakes or green onion, if desired. Enjoy!

This chopped Asian salad has low carb fixings like shredded cabbage, carrots, chicken, peppers, and crunchy peanuts. A smooth, creamy dressing with peanut butter and sesame oil adds rich flavor and a bit of spiciness.

INGREDIENTS

Salad Fixings:

- 1 (8-ounce) package raw coleslaw mix (Note 1)

- 3 cups shredded cooked chicken (Note 2)

- 5 scallions, thinly sliced (Note 3)

- 1 red bell pepper, cored, very thinly sliced lengthwise then cut in half widthwise

- 1 jalapeño, very thinly sliced widthwise or diced (Note 4)

- 1/2 cup roasted peanuts, roughly chopped

Peanut Dressing:

- 1/2 cup creamy peanut butter (Note 5)

- ◻ 1/4 cup toasted sesame oil (Note 6)

- ◻ 1/4 cup rice vinegar

- ◻ 1/4 cup water

- ◻ 1 tablespoon sriracha

- ◻ 1 teaspoon table salt

INSTRUCTIONS

Add all salad fixings to large bowl, big enough for tossing them. Set aside.

Make Dressing: In medium microwave-safe bowl or measuring glass, add all peanut dressing ingredients except for sesame oil. Microwave uncovered until peanut butter is just softened, about 15 seconds at high power (Note 7). Whisk in sesame oil until very smooth and fully combined, about a minute.

Toss Salad: Pour peanut dressing over salad fixings, tossing salad until well-mixed.

CONCLUSION

Exactly what you eat is up to you, but for the diet to work, you need to follow some rules. Cut saturated fat to less than 7 percent of your daily calories—which means eating less high-fat dairy, such as butter, and ditching fatty meats like salami. Make sure you get no more than 200 milligrams of dietary cholesterol a day, or the amount in about 2 ounces of cheese. And to further drop your LDL cholesterol, add in plant stanols or sterols, which are found in vegetable oil and certain types of margarine. If you follow the diet correctly, you'll be eating lots of fruits, vegetables, whole grains, low-fat or nonfat dairy products, fish and poultry without the skin.

www.ingramcontent.com/pod-product-compliance
Lightning Source LLC
Chambersburg PA
CBHW071940120726
48001CB00005B/1971